Table of Contents

A common sexually transmitted infection marked by genital pain and sores.

Caused by the herpes simplex virus, the disease can affect both men and women.

Pain, itching and small sores appear first. They form ulcers and scabs. After initial infection, genital herpes lies dormant in the body. Symptoms can recur for years.

Medication can be used to manage outbreaks.

BREAKFAST

1. Easy Tacos

Prep Time: 5 Minutes

Cook Time: 15 Minutes

Servings: 8

Ingredients:

- 8 small flour tortillas, (6" diameter), or corn tortillas for gluten free
- 12 oz chorizo sausage, (casings removed if present) or bacon
- 8 large eggs
- ¼ cup milk, (skim or whole milk)
- ¼ tsp fine sea salt
- 2 Tbsp unsalted butter

Toppings:

- 1 cup shredded cheddar, or Mexican cheese blend
- 1 large avocado, diced

- 1 cup Roasted Tomato Salsa, Pico De Gallo, or diced fresh tomatoes
- Hot sauce, to taste
- Cilantro, to garnish

Instructions

1. Preheat oven to 300°F and prepare all of the toppings so they are ready for assembly when the eggs are warm and ready.

Heat Tortillas:

2. Wrap flour tortillas in foil in 2 stacks of 4 and place in a preheated oven at 300°F for 15 minutes or until heated through. Remove from the oven and keep tortillas in foil to keep warm until ready to assemble. If using corn tortillas, toast on a dry cast iron skillet.

Cook Chorizo or Bacon:

3. Set a large skillet over medium/high heat and add chorizo. Break it up with a spatula and cook until browned and fully cooked through then transfer to a paper towel-lined plate to drain. If using bacon, cook bacon in the oven or make Air Fryer bacon until

browned and crisp then drain on paper towels and chop.

How to Scramble Eggs:

4. In a medium mixing bowl, add 8 eggs, ¼ cup milk and ¼ tsp salt, and beat together with a fork until eggs are well blended.

5. Place a large non-stick skillet over medium/low heat. Melt in 2 Tbsp butter. Once eggs are frothy, add well-beaten eggs. Let eggs sit for a moment until you see them starting to cook at the edges and bottom. Use a silicone spatula to pull the cooked eggs toward the middle, letting the liquid eggs take the place of the cooked eggs and working around the skillet as you go.

6. Towards the end, fold eggs onto themselves, but don't over-stir. Remove from the heat when the eggs still look a little moist and they will finish cooking on the residual heat from the skillet. Be careful not to overcook. When done, they should look moist, but not wet. Cover to keep warm until ready to assemble.

To Assemble Breakfast Tacos:

1. Fill each tortilla with eggs then shredded cheese to melt over the eggs. Add bacon or chorizo, avocado, pico or

salsa, and hot sauce if using along with your favorite toppings. Garnish with cilantro.

Prep Time: 3Minutes

Cook Time: 7Minutes

Servings: 1

Ingredients:

- 1 flour tortilla, 8" in diameter
- 2 large eggs
- 1 Pinch salt and pepper
- 1/4 cup shredded cheese, (1 oz) Mexican cheese, medium cheddar or mozzarella

Select Your Meat/ Protein:

- 3 oz breakfast Sausage, 2 patties
- 2 slices ham, (2 oz) chopped
- 2 slices bacon, (2 oz), sliced

Instructions

1. Heat a non-stick pan over medium heat. Cook Sausage or Bacon until browned and cooked through then remove to a plate. If using cooked ham, you can heat it

up or just add it over the cheese in step 4. Wipe excess oil from skillet if needed. Reduce heat to low.

2. In a measuring cup, add 2 eggs with a pinch of salt and pepper, or add seasoning to taste. Beat with a fork. Add beaten eggs and swirl to spread evenly over the bottom of the pan. Cook over low heat until when eggs are nearly cooked through (if you tilt the pan they shouldn't run).

3. Sprinkle the top with 2 Tbsp shredded cheese then cover with a tortilla. The cheese will make the tortilla stick to the egg. Use a large spatula to get under the egg and quickly flip over.

4. Sprinkle another 2 Tbsp of cheese or add cheese to taste. Sprinkle your cooked protein (sausage, bacon or ham) over half of the surface and fold the tortilla in half. Sautee on both sides until golden brown. Remove from skillet and use a pizza cutter to cut quesadilla into wedges and serve warm.

Prep Time: 10Minutes

Cook Time: 1hr 2Minutes

Servings: 10

Ingredients:

- 3 very ripe bananas, (medium/large)
- ½ cup unsalted butter, (8 Tbsp) at room temperature
- 3/4 cup granulated sugar
- 2 large eggs, lightly beaten
- 1 ½ cups all-purpose flour
- 1 tsp baking soda
- ½ tsp salt
- ½ tsp vanilla extract
- 1 cup walnuts
- ½ cup raisins

Instructions

1. Preheat the oven to 350°F. Grease and flour a bread loaf pan (9.25 long x 5.25 wide x 2.75 deep). Lightly roast walnuts on a skillet, continuously stirring so they

won't burn. Coarsely chop and cool to room temperature.

2. In a mixing bowl, cream together 8 Tbsp softened butter and 3/4 cup sugar (or honey if using honey).

3. Mash bananas with a fork until the consistency of chunky applesauce and add them to the batter along with 2 eggs, mixing until blended.

4. In a separate bowl, whisk together: 1 1/2 cups of flour, 1 tsp of baking soda and 1/2 tsp of salt then add to batter.

5. Add 1/2 tsp of vanilla extract and mix in chopped walnuts and raisins. Pour into prepared loaf pan. Bake at 350°F for 55-60 min or until a toothpick inserted into the center comes out clean. Let banana bread rest for 10 min before transferring to a wire rack to cool.

Prep Time: 10 Minutes

Cook Time: 30 Minutes

Servings: 5

Ingredients:

For the Shakshuka:

- 1 Tbsp olive oil
- 1/2 lb breakfast sausage
- 4 Tbsp unsalted butter
- 1 medium onion, (1 cup chopped)
- 28 oz canned whole peeled tomatoes, with their juice
- 1/2 tsp salt
- 1/4 tsp sugar
- 4 garlic cloves, (1.5 Tbsp minced)
- 1/4 cup parsley, finely chopped
- 5 large eggs

To Serve (optional):

- Parmesan grated over the top to serve
- Sliced Bread, buttered and toasted on a skillet

Instructions

1. Place a large 12-inch non-reactive skillet over medium heat, add 1 Tbsp olive oil and breakfast sausage. Sauté 5 minutes or until browned, breaking it up with a spatula, then transfer to a plate.

2. Melt in butter, add diced onion and sauté 4-5 minutes until soft and golden. Add garlic and stir another 30 seconds.

3. Add tomatoes with their juice and roughly break up the tomatoes with a spatula. Stir in 1/2 tsp salt and 1/4 tsp sugar to the pan, reduce heat and simmer uncovered for 15 minutes, stirring occasionally and breaking up the tomatoes into smaller pieces. Simmer until tomatoes are no longer watery but saucy and thick enough to create wells for the eggs.

4. Crack in 5 eggs into wells and lightly sprinkle salt on each egg.

5. Sprinkle cooked sausage around eggs then top with parsley. Cover and simmer on low heat 5-8 min (depending on desired doneness – check at 5 min) or until whites are cooked through and yolks are still soft and moist. Remove from heat and serve with freshly grated parmesan and toasted bread.

Prep Time: 15Minutes

Cook Time: 15Minutes

Servings: 4

Ingredients:

- 6 large eggs
- 1/3 cup heavy whipping cream
- 1/2 tsp salt, adjust to taste
- 1 cup grated mozzarella cheese
- 1/2 cup goat cheese
- 1/2 cup cherry tomatoes
- 1/2 cup bell pepper, red, orange or yellow
- 1 cup arugula
- 1 tbsp unsalted butter
- 1 tsp fresh herbs, for garnish

Instructions

1. Preheat the oven to 400F. Whisk eggs, heavy cream and salt until you get a smooth and even texture. Set aside.

2. Cut tomatoes in half. Chop bell peppers into small pieces.

3. Melt butter and coat the sides of the baking dish with it. Spread vegetables evenly on the bottom of the pan.

4. Pour over the egg mixture. Sprinkle the cheese on top. Using a fork, distribute the cheese around a little to incorporate it into the eggs. Bake for 15 to 17 minutes, or until the edges are set and the top is lightly browned.

Prep Time: 10Minutes

Cook Time: 50Minutes

Servings: 8

Ingredients:

- Cranberry Bread Ingredients
- 1 1/2 cups all-purpose flour
- 1 tsp baking powder
- 1/4 tsp salt
- 1/4 cup milk, room temperature
- Zest of 1 large orange, divided
- 1/4 cup orange juice, freshly squeezed
- 6 Tbsp unsalted butter, softened
- 3/4 cup granulated sugar
- 2 large eggs, room temperature
- 1 1/2 cups fresh cranberries, rinsed and patted dry
- 1/2 Tbsp all-purpose flour

Orange Glaze Ingredients:

- 1 cup powdered sugar

- 1 1/2 Tbsp freshly squeezed orange juice, or to reach desired consistency
- 1 tsp orange zest, reserved from the orange above

Instructions

How to Make Cranberry Orange Bread:

1. Prep: Preheat oven to 350°F. Butter a 6 cup (8 1/2 by 4 1/2 bread loaf pan) then dust with flour, tapping out the excess flour.
2. In a medium mixing bowl, whisk together: flour, baking powder, and salt. Set aside.
3. In a measuring cup, combine together milk, zest of 1 orange (Reserve 1 tsp zest for the glaze), and orange juice. Set aside.
4. In a large mixing bowl, cream together butter and granulated sugar on medium/high speed (2-3 minutes on high speed). It won't be smooth, just combined. Beat in 2 large eggs, mixing until well incorporated.
5. Add flour mixture in 2 parts, alternating with the milk mixture and mixing on medium/low speed just until incorporated with each addition. Scrape the sides of the bowl with a spatula as needed.

6. Toss cranberries with 1/2 Tbsp flour then fold them into the batter just until incorporated. Spread the batter into your prepared pan and bake for 45-50 min at 350°F until golden on top and a toothpick inserted into the center comes out clean. Let cool in pan 10-15 minutes then run a cake release tool or knife around the edges and transfer the loaf to a wire rack to cool completely before glazing.

Prep Time: 10Minutes

Cook Time: 45Minutes

Servings: 6

Ingredients:

- 6 medium baking apples,
- 1/2 cup brown sugar
- 1 tsp cinnamon
- 1/8 tsp grated nutmeg
- 1/3 cup dried cranberries, (craisins or raisins)
- 3 Tbsp unsalted butter
- 1/4 cup walnuts, finely chopped, optional
- 1 cup hot water

To serve (Optional):

- Unsweetened whipped cream or vanilla ice cream
- Caramel Sauce, (Try our recipe for easy homemade Caramel Sauce)

Instructions

1. Preheat oven to 375°F. In a small bowl, combine 1/2 cup brown sugar, 1 tsp cinnamon and 1/8 tsp nutmeg and stir with a fork. Stir in 1/3 cup dried cranberries and set aside.

2. Wash and core the apples using a melon baller, or small paring knife, leaving the base intact to keep the filling in – don't cut all the way through! Place apples in a casserole dish just big enough to hold the apples without them touching.

3. Divide the filling evenly between apples. Top each stuffed apple with 1/2 Tbsp butter, top with walnuts if using, and sprinkle with any remaining cinnamon mixture. Set apples into a 9×13 or 9×12 casserole dish.

4. Pour 1 cup hot water into the casserole dish and bake at 375°F for 45 minutes to 1 hour or until apples are soft (but not mushy). Baking time can vary by the type and size of apples you are using. My Jonagold apples (pictured here) were perfect after 45 minutes but I've had larger Braeburn apples take 1 hour.

Prep Time: 15Minutes

Cook Time: 20Minutes

Servings: 7

Ingredients:

For the Batter:

- ½ cup lukewarm water
- 1 cup milk
- 4 large eggs
- 4 Tbsp unsalted butter, melted. Plus more to sauté.
- 1 cup all-purpose flour, you can use 1/2 cup whole wheat flour and 1/2 cup all-purpose
- 2 Tbsp sugar
- Pinch salt

For the filling:

- 8 oz package cream cheese, at room temperature
- 16 oz small curd cottage cheese
- 1/4 cup sugar
- 1/2 cup raisins
- Powdered sugar for serving, optional

Instructions

How to Make the Crepes:

7. Put all of the ingredients for the crepes (in the order that they are listed) 1/2 cup warm water, 1 cup milk, 4 large eggs, 4 Tbsp melted butter, 1 cup flour, 2 Tbsp sugar and a pinch of salt in a blender and blend until well combined.

8. Melt a dot of butter in a non-stick skillet over medium heat (2 skillets make the process go faster).

9. As you are pouring into the skillet, swirl the batter to evenly coat the bottom. If you get any small gaps, you can fill them with more batter. Depending on the size of your skillet; add about 2-3 tbsp of batter. I use a small ladle.

10. Once the bottom is lightly golden (about a minute or less) flip the crepe using a sharp edged spatula to easily get under the crepe. Let the other side get lightly golden and plop the crepe out onto a cutting board. Repeat with remaining batter; you may not need to dot with butter after the first time if your skillet is a good one (and remember there is butter in the batter). Don't stack hot crepes on top of each other. Once they are just warm or room temp, they can be stacked. Don't panic,

my first crepe never turns out nice so I wolf it down to conceal the evidence!

How to make cheese filling and complete nalesniki:

1. In a colander, rinse the cottage cheese with cold water and drain well. Mash the cream cheese, cottage cheese and sugar with a potato masher until well combined and creamy. Cottage cheese will still be a little lumpy.

2. Using a spatula, spread 2 generous Tablespoons of cheese filling on each crepe and sprinkle with about 10-15 raisins.

3. Roll the crepe into a log and cut in half. Refrigerate crepes that aren't being served. It keeps in the fridge for almost one week.

To Serve:

1. Melt about 1 tablespoon of butter in a skillet and sauté the rolled cheese crepes on medium heat until golden brown on both sides. They don't take long to sauté. Be careful not to burn them.

2. Dust with powered sugar (optional) and serve with sour cream or jam on the side.

Prep Time: 5Minutes

Cook Time: 20Minutes

Servings: 6

Ingredients:

- 3 large eggs
- 2 Tbsp granulated sugar
- 15 oz pumpkin puree, (I used Libby's 100% Pure Pumpkin)
- 3/4 cup low-fat buttermilk, or kefir
- 1/4 tsp salt
- 1 1/4 cups all-purpose flour
- 1 Tbsp baking powder
- 1 tsp ground cinnamon
- Extra light olive oil , to sautee (or coconut oil or butter)

Instructions

1. In a large mixing bowl, whisk together eggs and sugar until well blended.
2. Whisk in pumpkin puree, buttermilk, and salt.

3. In a separate bowl, sift together flour, baking powder and cinnamon then whisk your flour mixture into the pumpkin mixture.

4. Heat a large non-stick skillet or griddle over medium heat and add just enough oil to lightly coat the surface. Spoon batter into the pan (about 2 Tbsp per pancake) and sautee 2-3 min per side. Repeat with remaining batter, adding more oil as needed. Serve warm with maple syrup.

Prep Time: 5Minutes

Cook Time: 20Minutes

Servings: 6

Ingredients:

- 1 1/4 cup ricotta cheese, (14-15 oz will work)
- 3/4 cup low fat buttermilk, (or kefir)
- 3 large eggs
- 2 Tbsp granulated sugar
- 1 1/4 cups all-purpose flour, (5 1/2 oz)
- 1 Tbsp baking powder
- 1/4 tsp sea salt
- Zest of 1 lemon
- Olive oil or coconut oil to cook

Instructions

1. In a large mixing bowl, whisk together eggs and sugar until well blended.
2. Mix in ricotta cheese, buttermilk and salt and whisk until blended.

3. In a separate bowl, sift together flour and baking powder then whisk the flour mixture into the cheese mixture.

4. Stir in the zest of 1 lemon. If you let the batter rest for 10-30 minutes, the pancakes will be even fluffier.

5. Heat a large non-stick skillet or griddle over medium heat and melt in your oil. Spoon batter into the pan (about 2 Tbsp per pancake) and sautee 2-3 min per side. Repeat with remaining batter, adding more oil as needed.

Prep Time: 20Minutes

Cook Time: 5hrs 20Minutes

Servings: 8

Ingredients:

- 4 lb boneless pork roast
- 3 Tbsp fine sea salt, (or 2 1/2 tsp table salt)
- 1 Tbsp ground black pepper
- 1 tsp dried oregano
- 1 large onion, diced
- 5 garlic cloves
- 4 Tbsp lime juice, (from 2 limes)
- 1/2 cup orange juice, (from 2 oranges)
- 1 cup chicken broth
- 2 bay leaves

Instructions

1. Pat the pork dry with a paper towel. Combine salt, pepper and dried oregano and rub pork with the seasoning.
2. In the slow cooker, add chopped onion, garlic cloves, broth, lime juice, orange juice, and bay leaves.
3. Add the pork to the slow cooker. Cook on high for 5 hours or on low for 7-8 hours.
4. Remove the pork from the slow cooker. Shredded the pork with two forks. Keep the juice.
5. To get crispy edges, transfer the shredded pork to a baking sheet. Pour ½ cup of the juices on top of the meat and broil it for 5-7 minutes, or until golden brown.

Prep Time: 10 Minutes

Cook Time: 3 Minutes

Servings: 8

Ingredients:

- 20 oz tuna in water, (four, 5-oz cans), well drained.
- 1 medium onion, 1 1/3 cup finely diced
- 1 medium granny smith apple, seeded and diced
- 1 avocado, pitted, peeled and diced
- 3/4 cup real mayo, or added to taste
- 1/2 tsp fresh lemon juice, or to taste
- 1/2 cup sliced almonds or chopped walnuts, toasted
- 1/8 tsp black pepper, or to taste

Instructions

1. Toast nuts on a dry skillet until golden. Remove from heat and cool slightly.
2. To drain tuna, I open the lid then press it down firmly over the tuna to drain off as much water as I can

squeeze out. If your tuna is too wet, your salad will be wet.

3. Combine all ingredients in a large mixing bowl and add a pinch of black pepper and 1/2 tsp lemon juice, or to taste. Add mayo to taste.

Prep Time: 10Minutes

Cook Time: 20Minutes

Servings: 4

Ingredients:

- 8 slices of bread, cut 1/2" thick
- 12 slices bacon
- 2 large ripe tomatoes, thickly sliced
- 4 green lettuce leaves, rinsed and spun dry
- 1 large avocado, or 2 small avocados pitted, peeled and sliced.
- salt and black pepper, to taste

Sauce for BLT Sandwiches:

- 1/2 cup real mayonnaise
- 2 Tbsp sour cream
- 2 tsp yellow mustard

Instructions

1. Preheat oven to 400°F. Place bacon on a foil-lined baking sheet in a single layer. Bake 18 to 20 minutes or until browned and crisp then transfer to a paper towel-lined plate to cool.

2. In a small bowl, combine sauce ingredients and set aside.

3. Lightly butter both sides of the toast and toast on a dry griddle or skillet over medium-high heat just until golden brown.

4. Arrange 4 slices of bread on a cutting board and spread 1 Tbsp of sauce over each toast. Add lettuce then tomato, bacon, avocado. Sprinkle salt and pepper over the avocado.

5. Spread 1 Tbsp sauce over the remaining toasted bread and place over the sandwich, sauce side down. Cut in half if desired and serve.

Prep Time: 15 Minutes

Cook Time: 15 Minutes

Servings: 4

Ingredients:

- 1 carrot, peeled and julienned
- 1 red bell pepper, sliced into strips
- 1 Tbsp unsalted butter
- 2 Tbsp oil, divided
- 1 lb flank steak, thinly sliced
- 1/4 cup cornstarch
- Sauce Ingredients-
- 1 tsp fresh ginger, peeled and grated
- 4 garlic cloves, peeled and grated
- 1/3 cup brown sugar, (packed)
- 1/3 cup water
- 1/3 cup low-sodium soy sauce,
- 1 tsp Sriracha, or added to taste
- 1/3 cup green onions, thickly sliced (from 4 stems)

Instructions

1. Place beef slices in a bowl, add cornstarch and stir to completely coat.

2. In a bowl, combine the ingredients for the sauce and stir until well combined, set aside.

3. Julienne the carrot and pepper, slice the onions. Thinly slice the beef into bite-sized strips.

4. In a skillet, heat 1 Tbsp oil with 1 Tbsp butter over med/high heat. Add the carrot and peppers, saute to desired tenderness. Remove the vegetables from the skillet.

5. Add 1 Tbsp oil over high heat. Once hot, add the beef and cook about 2 minutes per side.

6. Add the vegetables back into the skillet with the green onion.

7. Pour the sauce and stir to combine. Turn heat to medium/low and cook until the sauce thickens, about 3 minutes.

Prep Time: 15 Minutes

Cook Time: 15 Minutes

Servings: 14

Ingredients:

- 4 cups shredded chicken, from 2 large chicken breasts, (16 oz by weight)
- 2 large eggs
- 1/3 cup mayonnaise
- 1/3 cup all-purpose flour
- 3 Tbsp fresh dill, finely chopped (or 1 Tbsp parsley)
- 3/4 tsp salt or to taste
- 1/8 tsp black pepper
- 1 tsp lemon zest, plus lemon wedges to serve
- 1 1/3 cups mozzarella cheese, shredded
- 2 Tbsp olive oil to saute, divided
- 1 cup Panko bread crumbs

Instructions

1. In a large mixing bowl, whisk together: 2 eggs, 1/3 cup mayo, 1/3 cup flour, 3 Tbsp dill, 1/2 tsp salt, 1/8 tsp black pepper and 1 tsp lemon zest.

2. Add in shredded chicken and 1 1/3 cups shredded mozzarella then stir until chicken is well coated in batter.

3. Cover the bowl and refrigerate the mixture at least 30 minutes (this will help with forming patties). Use a trigger release ice cream scoop to divide into 12-15 cakes then form into 1/2-inch thick patties. Dip both sides in Panko crumbs.

4. Place a large non-stick skillet over medium heat. Add 1 Tbsp olive oil and half of the chicken patties. Sauté for 3-4 minutes per side until golden brown, adding more oil as needed. Repeat with remaining patties.

5. As soon as patties are off the heat, sprinkle with salt and squeeze fresh lemon juice over the patties. Serve warm.

Prep Time: 30 Minutes

Cook Time: 15 Minutes

Servings: 8

Ingredients:

- 2 lb pizza dough
- 1 cup pizza sauce
- 1 cup pepperoni
- 1/2 cup salami
- 2 cups shredded mozzarella
- 1 cup ricotta cheese
- 2 tbsp oil
- 1/2 cup parmesan cheese

Instructions

1. Preheat the oven to 475 °F. Line the baking sheet with parchment paper or spray it with oil.
2. Divide the dough into 8 equally sized pieces. Roll each piece into a 1/4" thick circle.

3. Place the filling on half of each circle (pizza sauce, ricotta, pepperoni, salami and shredded mozzarella). Make sure to leave the edges clean to allow for sealing the calzone. Fold the side over the filling and crimp the edges.

4. Place calzones on a baking sheet, leaving space apart. Cut a small vent on the top of each calzone. Brush the tops with oil and sprinkle with parmesan cheese. Bake for 15 minutes or until golden brown.

Prep Time: 25 Minutes

Cook Time: 20 Minutes

Servings: 8

Ingredients:

- 2 Tbsp unsalted butter
- 1 cup onion, finely diced (from 1 medium onion)
- 2 cups carrots, (3 medium), sliced into thin rings
- 4 cups low sodium chicken broth
- 4 cups broccoli, (2 heads of broccoli), cut into small florets
- 1 tsp garlic powder
- 1 tsp sea salt, or to taste
- 1/2 tsp black pepper
- 1/4 tsp thyme
- 3 Tbsp all-purpose flour
- 1/2 cup heavy whipping cream
- 1 tsp dijon mustard
- 4 oz sharp cheddar cheese, (2 cups shredded), plus more to garnish
- 2/3 cup parmesan cheese, (mild) shredded

Instructions

1. Prep all of your ingredients before you start cooking. In a Dutch oven or medium soup pot, melt 2 Tbsp butter. Add onion and carrots and saute until onions soften (5 minutes).

2. Add 4 cups chicken broth, 1 tsp garlic powder, 1 tsp salt, 1/2 tsp black pepper, and 1/4 tsp thyme. Bring to a boil then add broccoli and reduce to a simmer, partially cover, and cook until broccoli is softened (10-12 minutes depending on the thickness of broccoli).

3. Remove 2 cups of vegetables with a strainer and set aside. Blend remaining soup in the pot with an immersion blender or puree in batches in a blender. Blend until smooth or your desired consistency.

4. In a separate small bowl, combine 1/2 cup cream with 3 Tbsp flour and whisk vigorously until smooth and no longer lumpy then blend in 1 tsp dijon. The mixture will be thick like frosting. Bring the blended soup back to a boil and whisk in the cream/flour mixture, whisking for 3 to 4 minutes until smooth and thickened.

5. Remove the soup from the heat. Stir in the cheeses then stir in the reserved cooked vegetables. Season with salt to taste and serve right away. Garnish with more cheddar if desired.

Prep Time: 10 Minutes

Cook Time: 15 Minutes

Servings: 6

Ingredients:

- 2 Tbsp olive oil
- 1 lb mushrooms, sliced
- 1 small onion, finely chopped
- 4 Tbsp unsalted Butter
- 3 Tbsp all-purpose flour, gluten free flour works well too
- 1 1/2 to 2 cups chicken broth, (low sodium)
- 4-6 Cups leftover turkey meat, torn into bite-sized pieces
- 1/2 tsp sea salt , or to taste
- 1/8 tsp ground black pepper, or to taste
- 1 Tbsp Parsley to garnish, optional

Instructions

1. Heat a large non-stick pan over medium heat. Add 2 Tbsp olive oil and diced onions and sauté until soft and golden (4-5 minutes, stirring frequently). Add mushrooms to the pan and sauté until soft and golden (5-7 min, stirring frequently). Remove mushrooms and onions from pan.

2. In the same hot pan (no need to wash it), add 4 Tbsp unsalted butter. Once melted, whisk in 3 Tbsp flour. Cook, whisking continually until roux is a golden brown (1 1/2 to 2 min) then whisk in 2 cups chicken broth. Bring to a simmer and season to taste (I added 1/2 tsp sea salt and a pinch of black pepper).

3. Add add mushrooms/onions back to the pan. Stir in turkey and heat until turkey is just heated through. Garnish with finely chopped parsley if desired.

Prep Time: 15 Minutes

Cook Time: 30 Minutes

Servings: 6

Ingredients:

- 1 Tbsp olive oil
- 1 medium onion, chopped
- 3 garlic cloves, minced
- 1 jalapeno pepper, seeded and diced
- 1 tsp ground cumin
- 1 tsp chilli powder
- 1 lb chicken breasts, (2 medium)
- 20 oz crushed tomatoes
- 32 oz chicken broth
- 14 oz black beans, drained and rinsed
- 14 oz corn, drained and rinsed
- 1/2 cup cilantro, chopped, divided (reserve 1/4 of it for garnish)
- 1 lime, juiced
- 1 tsp salt, or to taste

Homemade Tortilla Strips:

- 1/4 cup olive oil
- 8 corn tortillas , (6" tortillas)

Toppings:

- 1 large avocado, diced
- 1 lime, cut into wedges, to serve

Instructions

Tortilla Strips:

1. Preheat a pan with 1/4 cup oil over medium-high heat. Cut tortillas into thin strips and fry them in batches in the hot oil until crisp. Remove from the pan and allow them to drain on a paper towel. Repeat with remaining tortilla strips, adding more oil as needed then set aside.

Chicken Tortilla Soup:

2. Preheat a pot with oil over medium-high heat. Add chopped onion, garlic and chopped jalapeño and sauté until veggies soften.
3. Add whole chicken, corn, beans, chilli powder, cumin, crushed tomatoes, salt, ¼ cup of cilantro and chicken

broth. Bring to a boil and let simmer for at least 25 minutes.

4. Remove chicken from the pot and shred it using 2 forks. Add shredded chicken back to the soup and simmer another 5 minutes then add lime juice.

5. Serve the soup with some tortilla strips, pieces of avocado, fresh cilantro and lime wedges.

Prep Time: 4hrs 2 Minutes

Cook Time: 5 Minutes

Servings: 6

Ingredients:

- 4 Tbsp fresh lemon juice
- 2 Tbsp extra virgin olive oil
- 1 Tbsp honey, or sugar
- 1/2 tsp salt
- 1/8 tsp black pepper

Ingredients for Kale Salad:

- 1 bunch kale, (8 cups loosely packed) well rinsed
- 1 cup craisins, dried cranberries
- 1 small red onion, thinly sliced
- 1 apple, (I used a crisp fuji apple)
- 1 pear, (firm)
- 1 cup pecans, toasted on a dry skillet

Instructions

1. Combine all dressing ingredients and stir together until honey dissolves then set aside.

2. Rinse and strip kale leaves. Chop in bite-sized pieces. I rinse the chopped leaves a second time to ensure there isn't any dust hidden in the curly leaves then dry in a salad spinner.

3. Place kale in a salad bowl, top with 1 cup craisins and drizzle with dressing. Use hands to stir well and massage lightly until kale just starts to wilt. Cover and refrigerate 4 hours or overnight.

4. Before serving, add sliced apples, sliced pears, thinly sliced onions and toasted pecans. Toss to combine.

21. Easy Vegetable Soup

Prep Time: 15 Minutes

Cook Time: 45 Minutes

Servings: 8

Ingredients:

- 2 Tbsp olive oil
- 1 medium yellow onion, chopped
- 2 large carrots, chopped
- 1 cup chopped celery
- 28 oz canned diced tomatoes
- 60 oz vegetable broth, low-sodium
- 3 medium potatoes, diced
- 1 cup green beans, chopped
- 3 bay leaves
- 2 tsp salt, or to taste
- 1 tsp ground black pepper
- 1 cup frozen sweet corn
- 1 cup frozen sweet peas
- 1/2 cup green onions, chopped

- 1/4 cup fresh parsley, ch

Instructions

1. Preheat a heavy soup pot or Dutch oven over medium heat and add 2 Tbsp olive oil. Add chopped onions and carrots and saute for 6-8 minutes, stirring occasionally until golden.

2. Add celery, canned tomatoes (with juice), broth, potatoes, green beans, bay leaves, salt, and pepper. Bring it to a boil then reduce heat to a simmer and cook for 25 minutes.

3. Once the vegetables are tender, add corn, sweet peas, green onion, and parsley. Season with salt to taste and simmer for another 5-8 minutes. Remove from heat and serve warm

Prep Time: 15 Minutes

Cook Time: 15 Minutes

Servings: 4

Ingredients:

- 6 oz instant Ramen noodles, (two 3 oz packages), seasoning discarded
- 1 lb broccoli, cut into 6 cups florets
- 2 Tbsp olive oil, divided
- 1 lb flank steak, or top sirloin, thinly sliced
- 2 tsp sesame seeds, optional garnish
- 2 Tbsp chives, optional garnish
- Stir Fry Sauce Ingredients:
- 1 tsp fresh ginger, peeled and grated
- 3 cloves garlic, grated (2 tsp)
- 6 Tbsp low sodium soy sauce
- 1/2 cup warm water
- 3 Tbsp light brown sugar, packed
- 1 1/2 Tbsp corn starch
- 2 Tbsp sesame oil
- 1/4 tsp black pe

Instructions

1. Start by cooking ramen so it is ready when you need it. Fill a medium saucepan with water and bring to a boil. Add ramen noodles and cook 3 minutes, breaking them up with a spatula. Drain and rinse with cold water and set aside.

2. In a large measuring cup or bowl, combine all sauce ingredients and stir to dissolve the sugar.

3. Place a large heavy skillet over medium heat. Once skillet is hot, add 1 Tbsp oil, 6 cups broccoli and 2 Tbsp water. Cover with lid and sauté for 4 minutes, stirring occasionally until crisp tender. Transfer broccoli to a separate dish.

4. Increase to medium high heat and add 1 Tbsp oil. Add beef in a single layer and sauté 2 minutes per side or just until cooked through then reduce heat to medium low.

5. Re-stir the sauce if it has separated and add to the pan and simmer 3-4 minutes, stirring occasionally. It will thicken. Return broccoli to the pan along with the cooked noodles and stir or toss to combine and coat the noodles in sauce. Add 1 to 2 Tbsp water to the sauce to thin if desired. Serve garnished with sesame seeds and chives.

Prep Time: 5Minutes

Cook Time: 15Minutes

Servings: 4

Ingredients:

For the Salad:

- 8 hard-boiled eggs
- 2 Tbsp celery, finely chopped
- 3 Tbsp red onion, finely chopped
- 3 Tbsp dill, chopped
- 3 Tbsp chives, chopped

For the Dressing:

- 1/3 cup mayonnaise
- 2 tsp lemon juice
- 2 tsp Dijon mustard
- 1/2 tsp paprika
- 1/2 tsp salt
- 1/4 tsp ground pepper
- 1 garlic clove, minced

Instructions

1. Cook eggs and cool. Once cooled, peel and chop eggs (we like ours chunky) and place into a salad bowl.
2. Add finely chopped celery, red onion, dill and chives.
3. In a sparate bowl, combine ingredients for the dressing. Gently stir dressing into the egg salad until coated and serve.

Prep Time: 5hrs 2 Minutes

Cook Time: 30 Minutes

Servings: 15

Ingredients:

- 2 1/4 cups Luke warm water
- 1/2 Tbsp salt
- 1 1/2 Tbsp sugar
- 2 tsp active dry yeast
- 3/4 cup whole wheat flour
- 3/4 cup rye flour, if you don't have rye, sub with whole wheat flour
- 3/4 cup better for bread flour
- Plus 2 1/2 cups better for bread flour
- 2 Tbsp canola oil plus more to grease the counter and pan
- For the Garlic topping:
- 4 garlic cloves
- 2 Tbsp water
- 1 tsp salt
- 6-8 strips of bacon

- 4 Tbsp olive oil

Instructions

1. In a large kitchen aid mixer bowl, combine 2 1/4 cups warm water (about 100°F), 1 1/2 Tbsp sugar and 1/2 Tbsp salt; stir to dissolve.

2. Sift the 3/4 cup wheat flour, 3/4 cup rye flour and 3/4 cup better for bread flour with 2 tsp yeast into the salted water. Do not discard anything left in the sifter (it's the good stuff!); toss it into the batter. Whisk together until well blended. Let it rise in a warm room uncovered for 2 hours, stirring the batter about once every hour. It will be bubbly.

3. Using the dough hook attachment add 1/2 cup all-purpose flour until well blended, scraping down the bowl if needed. Blend in the rest of your flour (2 cups) a heaping Tbsp at a time, letting the dough dissolve the flour in between each spoon (this takes about 20 min).

4. Once all the flour is incorporated, add 2 Tbsp canola oil. Let mix for an additional 20 more minutes or until dough is no longer sticking to your bowl. Note: after you add the oil it will look like it's coming off the walls and then it will appear to get stickier, then towards the

end of your 20 minutes, it will actually stop sticking to the walls as it mixes. Just let it do it's thing and everything will work out ;). If it's still really sticking to the bowl around the 20 min mark, add another heaping Tbsp of better for bread flour. Remove dough hook and Let it rise in the bowl, uncovered, until double in volume (45 min)

5. Grease your bread pans, counter and fingers a little with the canola oil and transfer the dough onto the oiled counter

6. Pinch the dough in the center to form two sections with your hands. Divide each section again and again, and again until you have a total of 30 rolls. Grease your rimmed baking dishes lightly with oil. Place dough balls onto each pan about 1/2" apart into each prepared pan and let it rise on the counter or outside if it's warm until 2 1/2 times in volume (about 1 1/2 hours - note: it rises faster if its in a warm place ~100°F). Bake at 360°F for 30 minutes or until rolls are golden.

7. While the rolls are baking, make your garlic mix: press 4 cloves of garlic into a small bowl and mix with 1 tsp salt and 2 Tbsp water. Chop your bacon into small strips, then saute on a dry skillet until golden brown.

8. Transfer bacon and the garlic mixture into a large silver bowl, stir in 4 Tbsp olive oil and toss the rolls with the garlic and bacon until your rolls are shiny. Leave the rolls in the bowl and keep it uncovered until the rolls are cooled down. These rolls are crisp on the outside and so so soft on the inside. You'll love them! The next day, try making sandwiches out of them.

Prep Time: 30 Minutes

Cook Time: 15 Minutes

Servings: 12

Ingredients:

Cloverleaf Rolls:

- 3 Tbsp warm water, (115°F)
- 2 1/4 tsp active dry yeast, (1 packet yeast)
- 1 cup low-fat milk, warm (105-110°F)
- 5 Tbsp unsalted butter, melted or very soft, plus more for the pan
- 3 Tbsp granulated sugar
- 1 large egg, room temperature
- 1 tsp fine sea salt
- 3 1/2 cups bread flour, divided (add an extra 1/4 cup if needed)

For the Topping:

- 3 Tbsp unsalted butter, divided, melted
- 1 tsp kosher salt

Instructions

1. In the bowl of a stand mixer, add 3 Tbsp very warm water (115°F). Sprinkle the top with 1 packet of yeast, whisk to combine, and let rest uncovered for 7 minutes until foamy on top.

2. Add warm milk, melted butter, sugar, egg, and salt. Whisk until blended, then gradually whisk in 2 cups of flour then switch to the dough hook attachment and add the remaining 1 1/2 cups of flour in thirds, letting it incorporate with each addition. Add more flour a little bit at a time until the dough feels moist to the touch, but it shouldn't stick to clean/dry fingertips.

3. Knead 10 minutes on speed 2 of a stand mixer, or knead by hand. The dough should pull away from the sides of the bowl as it kneads and will be smooth and elastic.

4. Transfer dough to a large oiled bowl, turning the dough to coat in oil. Cover the bowl with plastic wrap and let rise in a warm place (90-100°F) for 1 to 1 1/2 hours or until doubled in volume.

5. Transfer dough to a smooth, clean work surface. You should not need any additional flour at this point. Divide the dough into 12 even pieces then divide each piece of dough into 3 small pieces. Cup your hand over

each of the small pieces and roll over work surface to form a ball. Butter a 12-count muffin pan and place 3 little balls of dough into each muffin cup.

6. Oil a sheet of plastic wrap and place the oiled side loosely over the rolls. Let rest in a warm place for 30-45 minutes until visibly puffed. Meanwhile, preheat the oven to 425°F with a rack in the center.

7. Once rolls have risen, brush the tops with 2 Tbsp melted butter and bake in a preheated oven at 425°F for 13-15 minutes or until golden brown. As soon as they are out of the oven, brush with more melted butter and sprinkle with kosher salt. Transfer to a wire rack to cool for 15 minutes and serve warm.

Prep Time: 15 Minutes

Cook Time: 25 Minutes

Servings: 15

Ingredients:

- 1 1/2 cup whole milk, warmed to 110F
- 4 Tbsp unsalted butter, melted
- 1 Tbsp active dry yeast
- 1/3 cup granulated sugar
- 1 1/4 tsp salt, (we used fine sea salt)
- 4 cups all-purpose flour, (minus 1 to 3 Tbsp) measured correctly
- 1 Tbsp unsalted butter, melted to brush the tops of dinner rolls
- 1/2 tsp kosher salt, to sprinkle finished ro

Instructions

1. In the bowl of your mixer, whisk together warm milk (about 110F) and 1 Tbsp sugar. Sprinkle the top with 1 Tbsp yeast and let sit 1 minute. Whisk together and let

it sit for about 5 minutes until yeast looks foamy. Add 4 Tbsp melted butter, remaining sugar and salt.

2. Add flour half a cup at a time until the dough whisking to incorporate. Once the dough gets too thick, switch to the dough hook attachment and mix on speed 2 (you can also continue mixing by hand with a stiff spatula). Add about 4 cups of flour, adding the last 1 to 3 Tbsp of flour only if needed. The dough should feel sticky and tacky but should not stick to clean/dry finger tips.

3. Knead the dough with the dough hook in a stand mixer for 2 minutes or knead by hand (10 min), then place dough in an oiled bowl. Cover it with plastic wrap and let it rise about 2 hours in a warm place or until doubled in size.

4. Once the dough rises, turn it out onto a lightly floured surface and cut it into 15-24 even pieces depending on the shape of your baking dish. Roll each piece of dough into a ball and place them onto an oiled 9×13 casserole dish or baking sheet.

5. Cover the dinner rolls with plastic wrap and let them rise another 30-60 minutes in a warm place or until puffed (do not over-proof). Bake at 375F for about 23-25 minutes or until the tops are golden brown.

6. Immediately brush tops of dinner rolls with melted
    butter and set aside to cool to room temperature before
    serving

Prep Time: 10 Minutes

Cook Time: 20 Minutes

Servings: 4

Ingredients:

- 1 small onion, finely chopped
- 1/2 small green bell pepper, seeded and finely diced
- 1 Tbsp Worcestershire sauce
- 1 tsp yellow mustard
- 1/4 cup water
- 1 Tbsp brown sugar
- 15 oz can tomato sauce
- 1 lb lean ground beef, 85%-90% lean
- 1 Tbsp olive oil
- ½ tsp salt, or to taste
- ¼ tsp ground black pepper, or to taste
- 3 garlic cloves, minced
- 4 hamburger buns, toasted if desired

Instructions

1. Finely chop the onion. Seed and finely dice the green pepper.

2. In a bowl, combine the Worcestershire sauce, mustard, water, brown sugar, and tomato sauce.

3. Place a large skillet or Dutch oven over medium/high heat. Add olive oil and ground beef. Saute the beef for about 5 minutes until cooked through and longer pink, breaking it up with a spatula. Season with salt and pepper and add in the diced peppers and onion. Cook another 5 minutes until the veggies are tender and beef is browned.

4. Add the minced garlic and saute 30 seconds until fragrant, stirring constantly. Add in the sauce and bring to a light boil. Reduce heat to low and simmer uncovered for about 10 minutes. Season to taste with salt and pepper and serve on toasted buns for Sloppy Joe Sandwiches.

Prep Time: 18 Minutes

Cook Time: 12 Minutes

Servings: 16

Ingredients:

- 1 Tbsp olive oil
- 2 Tbsp unsalted butter
- 1 large or 2 medium yellow onions, thinly sliced
- 1/4 tsp sugar
- 1 oz au jus mix, made according to package instructions
- 3 cups water, to make the sauce, or to taste
- 16 Hawaiian sweet rolls
- 1/4 cup mayonnaise, thinly sliced
- 1 lb deli pastrami or roast beef, thinly sliced
- 9 slices mild provolone cheese, not aged
- 2 Tbsp unsalted butter, melted, plus more to grease baking sheet
- 1 Tbsp sesame seeds

Instructions

1. Preheat oven to 350°F. Butter a rimmed baking sheet.

2. Place a large skillet over medium/high heat with 1 Tbsp olive oil and 2 Tbsp butter. Add sliced onion and Sauté over medium heat for 5 minutes until softened, stirring occasionally. Sprinkle with 1/4 tsp sugar and sautee uncovered 5 minutes until caramelized and golden, stirring often. Transfer to a plate.

3. In the same pan, add 2 1/2 cups water and scrape the pan to deglaze. Add the au jus seasoning (adding to taste*) then bring to a boil, reduce heat and simmer according to package instructions. Add more water to taste if it's too salty.

4. Cut buns in half. Place the bottom half of dinner rolls on a buttered baking sheet and spread 1/4 cup mayo. Layer folded slices of beef evenly over the rolls. Spread caramelized onions over your sliders. Cover the beef with sliced provolone.

5. Place the top of buns over and brush the tops with 2 Tbsp melted butter then immediately sprinkle tops with sesame seeds. Bake uncovered at 350°F for 12-15 minutes, or until cheese is melted and tops are golden brown.

6. Cut through the buns with a serrated knife to separate into individual sliders. Serve with warm au jus dip.

Prep Time: 30 Minutes

Cook Time: 50 Minutes

Servings: 12

Ingredients:

- 1 lb ground beef, (15-20% fat content)
- 1 medium onion, finely diced
- 2 large garlic cloves, minced
- 1/4 cup dry red wine, or beef broth
- 1 Tbsp olive oil
- 24 oz Marinara Sauce , (3 cups)
- 1/2 tsp sea salt
- 1/4 tsp black pepper, ground
- 1/4 tsp dried thyme
- 1/2 tsp granulated sugar
- 2 Tbsp parsley, finely chopped
- 9 lasagna noodles, cooked al dente

Ingredients for Cheese Sauce:

- 16 oz low-fat cottage cheese
- 15 oz reduced fat ricotta cheese

- 1 large egg
- 2 Tbsp parsley, finely chopped, plus more to garnish
- 4 cups mozzarella cheese, shredded, divided

Instructions

How to Make Meat Sauce:

1. Place a deep pan or Dutch oven over medium/high heat and add 1 Tbsp olive oil, 1 lb ground beef and diced onion. Saute, breaking up the meat, for 5 minutes or until beef is no longer pink. Add pressed garlic and sauté another minute until fragrant.
2. Add 1/4 cup wine and stir for 2 minutes or until wine is nearly evaporated. Add 3 cups marinara, 1/2 tsp salt, 1/4 tsp pepper, 1/4 tsp thyme, 1/2 tsp sugar and 2 Tbsp parsley. Bring to a simmer then cover and cook 5 minutes.

How to Make Cheese Sauce:

1. In a large mixing bowl, combine 16 oz Cottage Cheese, 15 oz Ricotta, 1 cup mozzarella, 1 egg and 2 Tbsp parsley. Mix well.
2. How to Make Lasagna:

3. Preheat oven to 375°F. Bring a large pot of water to a boil. Add salt and 9 lasagna noodles. Cook until al dente according to package instructions.

4. Spread 1/2 cup meat sauce in the bottom of a deep 9×13 casserole dish. Add 3 noodles, spread on 1/3 of the meat sauce, and sprinkle with 1 cup mozzarella cheese. Spoon on and spread the top with 1/2 of your cheese sauce.

Repeat until you have 3 layers of noodles:

1. Add 3 noodles, 1/3 meat sauce, 1 cup mozarella cheese, 1/2 cheese sauce

2. Add 3 noodles, remaining 1/3 meat sauce, remaining 1 cup mozarella.

3. Poke 9-12 toothpicks over the surface of your lasagna (to keep the foil from sticking to the cheese). Cover with foil and bake at 375°F for 45 minutes.

4. Remove foil and broil for 3 to 5 minutes, or until cheese turns golden. Let lasagna rest 30 min before slicing.

Prep Time: 8 Minutes

Cook Time: 22 Minutes

Servings: 24

Ingredients:

- 2 lb lean ground beef, (90/10 or 93/7 fat content)
- 1/2 Tbsp olive oil
- 1 tsp salt
- 1 tsp black pepper
- 1 tsp garlic powder
- 1/2 large yellow onion, finely diced
- 1/4 cup mayonnaise
- 8 slices medium cheddar cheese
- 6 oz medium cheddar, shredded (or used more sliced cheese)
- 24 dinner rolls, (or use 2 packs of 12)
- 2 Tbsp unsalted butter, melted, plus more to grease baking sheet
- 1 Tbsp sesame see

Instructions

1. Preheat oven to 350°F. Butter the bottom of a rimmed baking sheet.

2. Place a large skillet over medium/high heat with 1/2 Tbsp olive oil. Add diced onion then 2 lbs ground beef and break up with a spatula. Season with 1 tsp salt, 1 tsp black pepper, and 1 tsp garlic powder. Sautee over medium/high heat, breaking up the beef and cook just until cooked through then remove from heat.

3. Tilt skillet to spoon off and discard excess fat. Stir in 1/4 cup mayo.

4. Cut buns in half. Place bottom half of dinner rolls on buttered baking sheet and line bread with sliced cheese. Spread ground beef mixture evenly over the sliced cheese, using the back of a spatula to square off the edges. Cover the ground beef with 6 oz of shredded cheddar.

5. Place the top of buns, cut-side down, over the burgers. Brush tops with 2 Tbsp melted butter and immediately sprinkle tops with sesame seeds. Bake at 350°F for 12-15 minutes, or until cheese is melted and tops are golden brown.